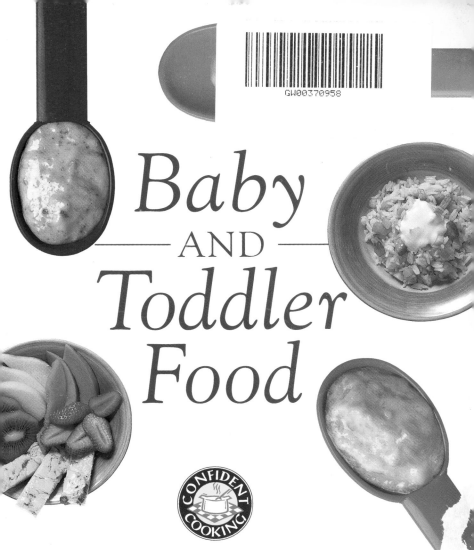

Baby
— AND —
Toddler
Food

This book has been produced in accordance with the guidelines set out by the
Adelaide Women's and Children's Hospital "Safe Eating for Young Children"
project. To help prevent the dangers of choking, do not give young children food
that can break off in hard pieces, such as raw carrot, celery or apple (these should
be grated or cooked), and avoid nuts, popcorn, cornchips and hard lollies.

MURDOCH BOOKS®
Sydney • London • Vancouver • New York

COOKING FOR YOUR CHILD

Preparing quick, nourishing meals for your baby or toddler is not difficult, even for a busy mother.

Sometimes the thought of preparing food for a baby about to be weaned from breast or bottle can be very daunting—particularly if cooking isn't really one of your great talents. But with a little thought and planning, nourishing tasty food is not difficult to achieve, even for the first-time mother (and cook).

Commercial baby foods are designed to be convenient and they are just that. They are not intended to replace every meal. They lack the texture necessary to stimulate chewing skills, don't help your baby learn about taste and flavour and, above all, can prove expensive.

After up to six months of thriving on breast or bottle milk, you will begin to notice that your baby needs more food more often. Babies are individuals with differing needs, so there can be no hard and fast rules about this important step, but usually by four to six months you will begin experimenting with solid food. It is important not to introduce solid food too early as your baby's digestive system may not yet be ready.

When you feel that it is time for solid feeding to begin, usually around the fifth or sixth month, your baby may be growing quickly and be happy to receive the extra nourishment. But many babies still do not, at this stage, require more than milk alone. It will be a time of experimentation for both of you and if, after several attempts, your baby is not interested, delay it for another few weeks.

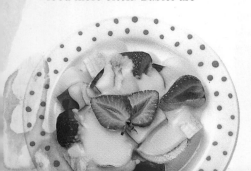

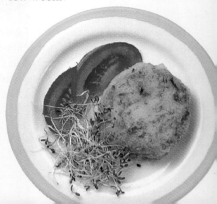

First solids should be nutritious to allow for normal, happy development and to help resist disease. Rice cereal is the traditional first food and gradually new tastes and textures are introduced. Try one at a time, in small amounts, even if your baby seems to love the taste. Allow for individual preferences and don't worry if at times your baby isn't interested in what you are offering—it isn't a criticism of your cooking. Remember, providing your baby is in good health, these meals are only a minor part of his daily diet, which will still consist mainly of milk. Your baby will enjoy and should be able to tolerate several different foods in the early weeks of spoon feeding. Well-ripened fruit, such as bananas, are easier to digest. Mashed with a fork and mixed with a little cereal or juice, they are perfect. Gradually increase the thickness and texture as your baby learns to chew.

Within two months of introducing solid foods, your child's consumption may have increased to as much as six or eight tablespoons of solids daily, including a number of different foods. By this time he may be enjoying three meals a day. Variety in the diet is not yet important. He would probably be content with the same foods at each meal. You can start selecting new foods to interest him, however.

When it comes to meal preparation for baby, the appliances that are helpful are the freezer, microwave and blender. It doesn't mean you have to run out and purchase any of these items (an ordinary potato masher can be used to purée soft food such as cooked pumpkin) but if you have them, use them.

Before you know it, your baby will be eating three meals a day along with the rest of the family and you'll be wondering where the time went. Introducing your child to solid food should be fun. Enjoying each new stage of your baby's development is all part of the joy of parenting.

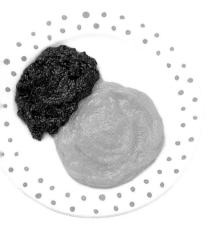

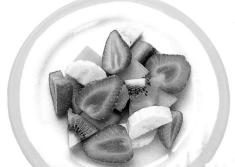

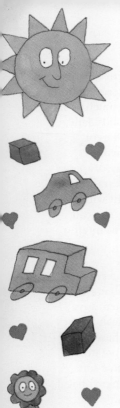

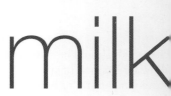

milk

Every mother makes an individual choice whether to breast or bottle feed her baby. It's an important question. The first weeks are the bonding time between mother and child and you need to relax and enjoy them together. Your decision is the right one.

■ Breast milk provides perfect nutrition and important substances which protect the baby against infection. The first fluid to come from the breasts is not milk, but it is just as important for your baby. It is a yellowish substance called colostrum, rich in antibodies and protein but with less sugar and fat than the milk that follows.

■ In the first three days after the birth, the mother's milk will be mainly colostrum. This changes to become normal milk over the next three to four days.

■ Milk production is stimulated by the baby sucking at the breast. The milk changes during the feed: the 'fore' milk at the beginning is thin and watery while the later 'hind' milk is richer in fat. Some babies settle better after being fed completely from one breast while others drain both sides.

■ There are no rules for how long and often your baby feeds— it may be every two to four hours around the clock. Allow him to drink for as long as he wants. Your midwife or early childhood nurse will reassure you as to whether your baby is gaining the right amount of weight.

■ You may worry that your baby is not receiving enough milk and consider topping up the breast milk with formula. This will decrease your breast supply, so is not a good idea unless you want to wean the baby from breast to bottle.

allergies

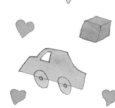

■ The foods which most commonly cause reactions include eggs (particularly egg whites), cow's milk, fish and peanuts. An allergy to cow's milk makes it impossible to wean a baby from breast to most formulas, as well as cow's milk. Soy bean milk may be the answer, but always consult your doctor.

■ Because of the danger of choking, don't give whole or chopped nuts to children under seven years.

■ Children tend to grow out of allergies to egg, milk, wheat and soy by the age of five or six, though sometimes a particular food such as fish or peanuts can cause problems for life.

■ If your toddler has a food allergy and is going to a party, ring the hosts beforehand and let them know what food your child cannot have. Give your toddler something to eat and drink before going to the party.

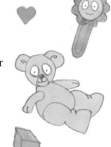

■ Make sure that anyone who may prepare or buy food for your child (grandparents, childminder) knows about an allergy.

■ Food intolerances are more common than food allergies and can occur at any time during life. They are due to small chemicals in foods which have a lot of natural or artificial flavour, such as sweets, cordial, fruit juice, strawberries, dried fruit, honey and chocolate.

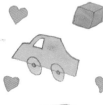

■ The amount of food chemicals can build up in the body from a variety of foods. Symptoms only occur when the total amount is higher than the child can tolerate. Symptoms vary from person to person, but may include irritability, hyperactivity, skin rashes, leg pains and headaches. To control symptoms, the quantity of problem foods will need to be reduced.

FIRST FOODS FOR BABIES 4–9 MONTHS

Cereal—easy to swallow and digest—is the traditional first food. All recipes serve one baby unless stated.

RICE CEREAL

Combine 1 teaspoon rice cereal with enough breast milk/formula or boiled water to produce a thick consistency.

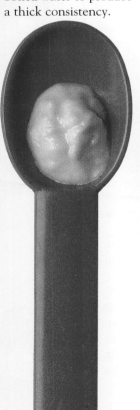

WEETBIX

Crush a quarter of a Weetbix and mix with a little breast milk, formula or boiled water to produce the desired consistency.

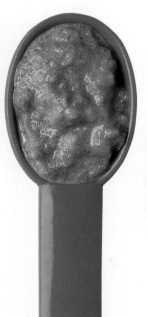

PORRIDGE

Combine 1 tablespoon rolled oats and 1 tablespoon cold water. Stir in 1 1/2 tablespoons hot water. Bring to the boil, stirring, and then reduce the heat and simmer for 1 minute. Purée with enough breast milk or formula to produce the consistency required.

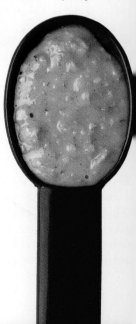

STEWED FRUIT

Peel, core and slice
1 apple, peach or pear
and put in a small pan
with 2 tablespoons
water. Bring to the
boil, reduce the heat
and simmer until soft
and pulpy, adding more
water as required. Purée
with a little boiled
water to make $^{1}/_{2}$ cup
of stewed fruit.

RICE CEREAL AND STEWED FRUIT

Combine 1 teaspoon
rice cereal with
1 teaspoon stewed fruit
or mashed banana. Add
enough breast milk,
formula or boiled water
to produce a soft, but
not runny, cereal.

BABY CEREAL WITH FRUIT AND YOGHURT

For older babies, mix
together baby cereal,
stewed fruit, baby
yoghurt and breast
milk, formula or boiled
water to produce the
desired consistency.

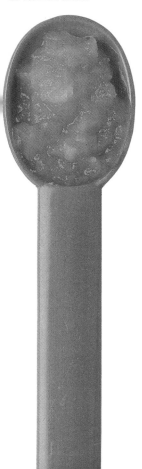
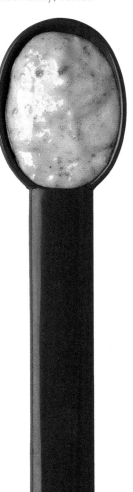
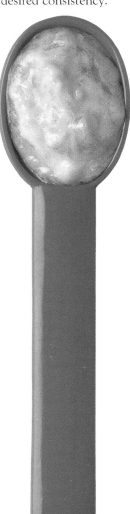

Ideas for purées
Always purée using breast milk, formula or boiled water.
∎ Mashed avocado and cottage cheese.
∎ Sieved tomato and avocado. Peel and seed the tomatoes before pressing them through a sieve. Peel tomatoes by cutting a cross in the top and plunging them into boiling water for 1 minute. Refresh in cold water and the skin will easily peel away. Quarter, then remove the seeds with a spoon.
∎ Mashed ripe banana and strained orange juice.
∎ Puréed apple, pear and banana.
∎ Cottage cheese and stewed fruit.
∎ Creamed potato.
∎ Puréed pumpkin.
∎ Puréed potato, pumpkin and zucchini.
∎ Puréed sweet potato and avocado.
∎ Puréed potato, baked beans and cottage cheese or grated mild cheese.
∎ Puréed spinach and cheese sauce.
∎ Puréed vegetable soup.
∎ Puréed vegetables and well-cooked meat.
∎ Puréed vegetables and cooked fish.

TOAST FINGERS
Butter 1 slice of toast and cut into fingers for an older baby.

HOME-MADE RUSKS
Remove the crusts from 5 thick slices of stale bread. Cut the bread into fingers or use shaped cutters. Put the bread on a baking tray and bake in a very slow oven (130°C) for about 1 hour or until dry and hard. Allow to cool thoroughly and store in an airtight container. Makes about 20 rusks.

PUREED VEGETABLES
Put $^1/_2$ cup peeled and chopped vegetables in a steamer basket over a saucepan of gently simmering water, cover tightly and steam until very tender. Purée with a little breast milk, formula or boiled water.

Note: Don't ever heat baby's milk or feeds in the microwave: some areas can become very hot while others remain cool.

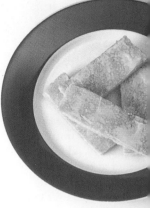

Clockwise from top left: *Toast Fingers; Cheese Sauce with vegetables; Vegetable Soup; Puréed Vegetables; Rusks*

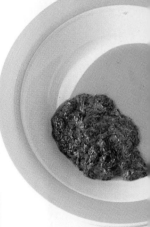

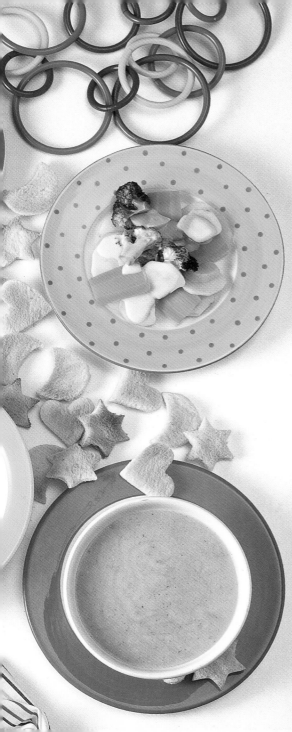

CHEESE SAUCE

Melt 15 g butter in a small saucepan. Mix in 2 teaspoons plain flour and cook for 1 minute, stirring continuously. Remove from the heat and gradually blend in $1/2$ cup milk until smooth. Return to the heat and stir continuously until the sauce boils and thickens. Reduce the heat and simmer for 2 minutes. Blend in 2 tablespoons grated mild Cheddar cheese. This makes about $1/2$ cup of sauce which you can serve with boiled or mashed vegetables, or bread.

VEGETABLE SOUP

Put 2 cups water in a pan with 1 cup chopped mixed vegetables and 1 tablespoon rice. Bring to the boil, reduce the heat and simmer until the vegetables and rice are tender. Allow to cool and then purée before serving. Freeze or refrigerate any leftovers. You can give older babies croutons.

TODDLER BREAKFASTS

For toddlers, as for adults, breakfast can be the most important meal of the day. All serve one unless stated.

CEREAL MIXTURES

Blend milk with rice cereal, yoghurt and stewed or chopped fresh or dried fruit. Put the dish in a bowl of hot water and stir until warmed. Alternatively, warm in the microwave on Medium (50%) power, for 45 seconds, blending in more milk as required. Always test the temperature before serving.

TODDLER MUESLI

Mix together
1 cup rolled oats,
1/2 cup mixed dried fruit (chopped or grated dried apple, apricot, pear or coconut),
2 crushed Weetbix and
2 tablespoons oat bran. Store in an airtight container. Serve with a little milk.

> **Note:** For fussy toddlers, add 1/2 cup rice bubbles, corn flakes or other favourite cereal.

FRUITY RICE

Mix together 1/2 cup warm, cooked rice and 1/4 cup chopped, fresh or dried fruit. Top with a dollop of natural yoghurt.

> **Note:** If your child is not yet chewing adequately, substitute puréed fruit for pieces. Flavoured yoghurt or yoghurt dessert can be used instead of natural yoghurt.

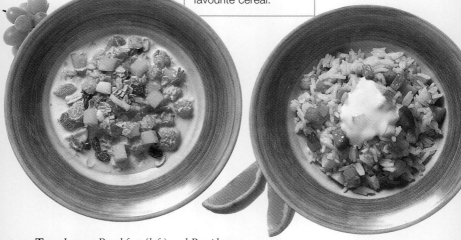

Top: *Instant Breakfast (left) and Porridge*
Below, from left: *Toddler Muesli; Fruity Rice; Fruit Mixtures; Cereal Mixtures*

INSTANT BREAKFAST

Rather than just pouring out a bowl of cereal, serve buttered slices of fruit bread and a mixture of sliced fresh fruit (kiwi, apple, pear, melon, strawberry) for a delicious instant breakfast.

PORRIDGE

Prepare porridge oats as directed on the packet, with water or milk. Add chopped fresh fruit, dried fruit, stewed fruit, honey or brown sugar, for a warming breakfast.

FRUIT MIXTURES

Combine stewed, chopped fresh or dried fruit with yoghurt. If you are using natural yoghurt, drizzle with a little honey.

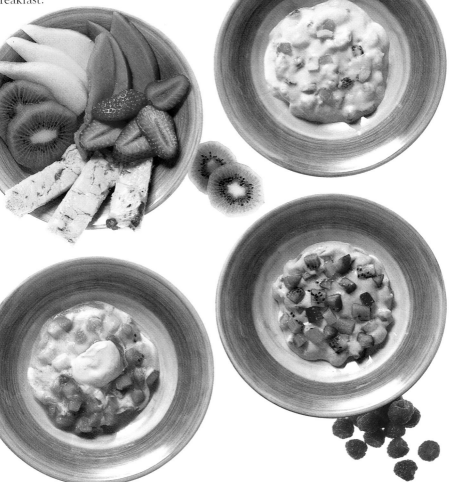

Toast Toppers

■ Toast 2 slices bread under a hot grill until golden on both sides. Sprinkle with $1/2$ cup grated mild Cheddar cheese and grill until the cheese melts. Slice into fingers. Toppings can be put on crumpets and muffins as well.

■ Top a slice of toast with a slice of tomato. Grill for about 1 minute and then sprinkle with grated cheese. Grill until the cheese melts and then slice into fingers.

■ Spread toast with mashed baked beans and sprinkle with grated cheese. Grill until the cheese melts and slice into fingers.

■ Mix together $1/2$ cup grated cheese with $1/2$ chopped tomato and 1 finely chopped slice of ham. Spread over a slice of toast and grill until the cheese melts. Slice into fingers.

■ Spread a slice of toast with mashed avocado. Sprinkle with grated cheese and grill until the cheese melts. Slice into fingers.

CHEESY EGGS

Melt 1 teaspoon butter in a small saucepan and cook 1 tablespoon peeled chopped tomato until tender. Whisk together 1 egg, 1 tablespoon milk and 1 tablespoon grated Cheddar cheese and add to the pan. Cook gently, stirring until thickened. Serve with toast or bread to toddlers who have started eating egg. Poached eggs are also easy and nutritious for toddlers. Poach in simmering water for 2–3 minutes.

BANANA SMOOTHIE

Put 1 cup milk, 2 tablespoons plain yoghurt and 1 small ripe banana in a food processor and process until smooth. Add a little honey or sugar to sweeten if you like. Serve immediately with a straw.

MILK SHAKE

Put 1 cup milk, $1/3$ cup vanilla yoghurt, 1 scoop vanilla ice cream and a few drops of vanilla essence in a food processor. Process until well combined and frothy. Serve immediately with a straw.

FRENCH TOAST

Beat an egg with a little milk. Cut a thick slice of white bread into squares and dip into the egg. Cook in a non-stick frying pan, brushed with a little oil or melted butter, until golden on both sides.

Clockwise from top left:
*Banana Smoothie;
Milk Shake; Fruity Dip;
French Toast; Cheesy Eggs*

FRUITY DIP

Pour $1/2$ cup flavoured yoghurt or yoghurt dessert into a serving dish. Grate or cut a variety of fruit into small pieces (banana, pear, apple, kiwi fruit, pawpaw, strawberries or whatever is in season). Serve with the yoghurt for dipping. You could use cottage cheese instead of yoghurt.

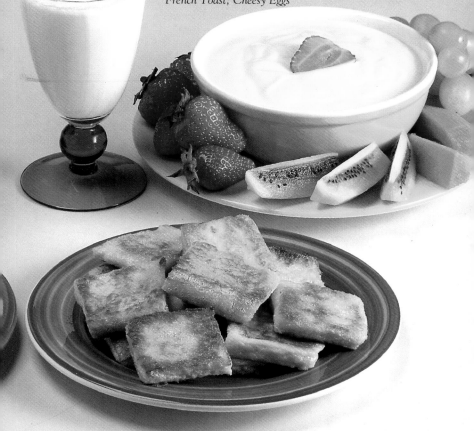

JUNIOR PIKELETS

Preparation: **10 minutes**
Cooking time: **20 minutes**
MAKES ABOUT **24**

1 cup self-raising flour
1/4 teaspoon
    bicarbonate of soda
2 tablespoons caster
    sugar
1 egg
1/2 cup milk
2 teaspoons oil
1/2 cup sultanas,
    optional

1 Sift the flour and
  soda together into a
bowl. Stir in the sugar.
2 Make a well in the
  centre and whisk in
the combined egg, milk
and oil to make a
smooth batter. Add the
sultanas for children
over 12 months old.
3 Heat and lightly
  grease a frying pan.
Drop teaspoons of the
batter into the pan and
cook until bubbles
form. Turn and cook
the other side until
golden. Cool on a wire
rack. Serve with butter.
Can be frozen, layered
between sheets of
greaseproof paper, for
up to 1 month.

MINI APPLE MUFFINS

Preparation: **10 minutes**
Cooking time: **15 minutes**
MAKES ABOUT **24**

2 cups plain flour
1 tablespoon baking
    powder
1 teaspoon ground
    cinnamon
1/2 cup brown sugar
1 cup milk
125 g butter, melted
1 egg, beaten
2 green apples, peeled,
    cored and grated

1 Preheat the oven to
  200°C. Sift the
flour, baking powder
and cinnamon into a
bowl. Stir in the sugar.
2 Make a well in the
  centre and add the
combined milk, butter,
egg and apple. Blend
together, stirring no
more than 15 times.
3 Spoon into greased
  mini muffin tins
until 3/4 full. Bake for
15 minutes, or until
cooked and golden.
Cool on a wire rack
and store in an airtight
container. Muffins can
be frozen in a sealed
bag for up to 1 month.

CHEESY BRAN MUFFINS

Preparation: **10 minutes**
Cooking time: **15 minutes**
MAKES ABOUT **24**

2 cups plain flour
1 tablespoon baking
    powder
1 cup grated Cheddar
    cheese
1/2 cup unprocessed
    bran
1 cup milk
125 g butter, melted
1 egg, beaten

1 Preheat the oven to
  200°C. Sift the flour
and baking powder into
a bowl. Stir in the
cheese and bran.
2 Make a well in the
  centre and add the
combined milk, butter
and egg. Fold together,
stirring no more than
15 times (the batter
will still be lumpy).
3 Spoon into greased
  mini muffin tins
until 3/4 full. Bake for
15 minutes, or until
golden. Cool on a wire
rack and store in an
airtight container.
Muffins can be frozen
in a sealed bag for up
to 1 month.

From top: *Junior Pikelets; Mini Apple Muffins;* ▶
Cheesy Bran Muffins

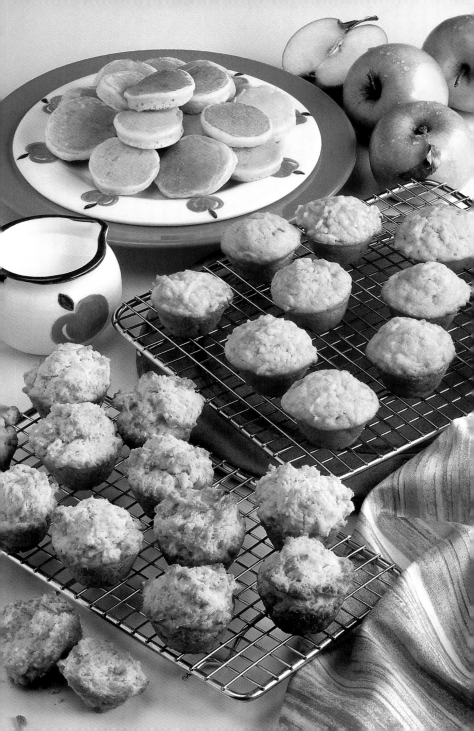

TODDLER LUNCHES

Lunchtime can be fun with these ideas for quick meals, so pull up a chair and enjoy your toddler's company.

SAUSAGE ROLLS

Preheat the oven to 200°C. Mix together 125 g sausage mince with 125 g minced steak, 1 tablespoon tomato sauce and 2 teaspoons plain flour. Form into a sausage shape. Place along one edge of a thawed sheet of ready-rolled puff pastry. Roll up and cut into short lengths. Place on a baking tray. Brush with a little milk or beaten egg. Bake for 15–20 minutes. Serve with salad.

QUICK AS A WINK PIES

Preheat the oven to 200°C. Place leftover savoury mince, meat casserole, bolognese sauce or sweet curry in the base of a small ramekin. Top with thawed, ready-rolled puff pastry (cut a small steam hole in the centre). Brush with milk or beaten egg and bake for 15–20 minutes. Cool to serve.

MY FIRST SALAD

Children love food they can eat with their fingers, so salads are ideal. Try crisp lettuce leaves topped with grated carrot, tomato wedges, slices of cheese or cold cooked meats, and orange segments or chunks of kiwi fruit. Hard foods like carrot or apple should be grated, not chopped, to prevent choking.

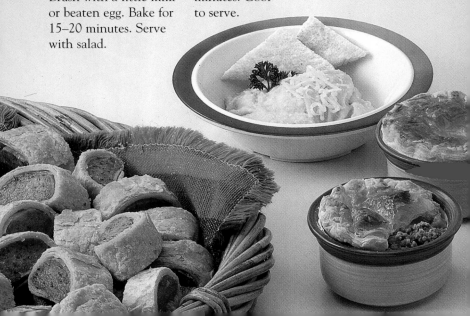

COTTAGE CHEESE AND CHICKEN

Mix together $1/2$ cup chopped cooked chicken, $1/2$ cup cottage cheese, half a tomato, chopped, and quarter of an avocado. Serve with bread and butter, toast fingers or pieces of roll. Alternatively, stir into cold, cooked pasta shells.

CHEESY BAKED BEANS

Peel and chop 1 potato and boil until very tender; drain. Add 130 g baked beans and $1/4$ cup grated mild Cheddar or cottage cheese. Purée or mash with a little milk and serve warm with bread and butter.

AVOCADO DIP

Mix together half an avocado, $1/4$ cup grated mild Cheddar cheese and quarter of a tomato, chopped. Purée or mash the mixture well. You could also add a few drops of French dressing. Serve with toast fingers.

From left: *Sausage Rolls; Cheesy Baked Beans; Quick as a Wink Pies; My First Salad; Cottage Cheese and Chicken; Avocado Dip*

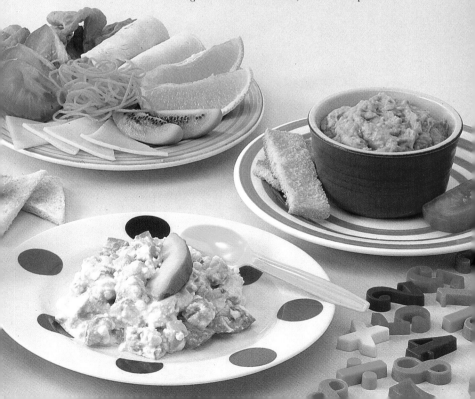

LOTS OF SANDWICHES

Use a variety of breads (such as lavash, pitta, rolls, bagels, wholemeal and so on) for making sandwiches and serve with milk or diluted fruit juice for a quick nutritious lunch. Try these ideas for fillings:

- ham and cheese
- egg and tomato
- taramasalata and lettuce
- hummus and bean sprouts
- cold cooked ham or chicken and tomato
- cold cooked rissoles or sausage with tomato sauce
- Vegemite, cheese and cucumber
- cottage cheese, grated carrot and avocado

BITS AND PIECES WITH DIP

Arrange small slices of cheese, cold cooked meat, salad vegetables such as seeded cucumber or chopped tomatoes, fruit and bread sticks on a plate. Serve with a quick and easy lunchtime dip such as yoghurt flavoured with mashed avocado, cottage cheese or hummus.

Note: It may be tempting for busy mothers, but never leave children alone while they are eating. Sticks of hard raw vegetables and fruit such as carrot or apple are only suitable for older children— they should be grated, cooked or mashed for younger children and toddlers. Always remove any skin and seeds which could cause choking. Make sure children sit quietly while they eat—running, playing, laughing or crying while eating can lead to choking.

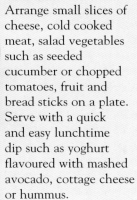

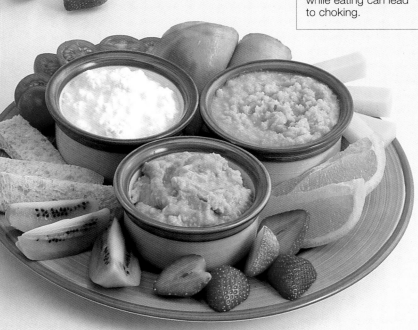

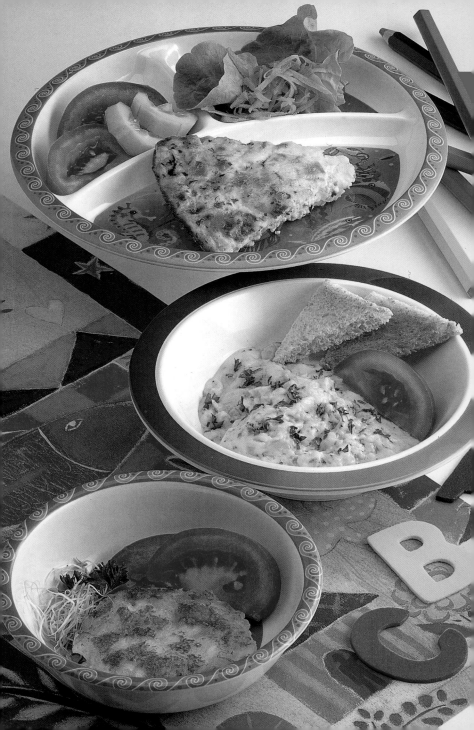

SAVOURY FLAN

Preparation: **15 minutes**
Cooking time: **45 minutes**
SERVES **8**

1 1/2 cups grated cheese
125 g ricotta cheese
125 g ham, chopped or
2 rashers rindless
    bacon, grilled and
    chopped
1 zucchini, grated
1 tablespoon chopped
    fresh parsley
3 eggs
1 1/2 cups milk

1 Preheat the oven to
    180°C. Mix together
the cheeses, ham or
bacon, zucchini and
parsley. Place in the
base of a greased 23 cm
flan dish or pie plate.

2 Whisk together the
    eggs and milk and
pour into the dish.

3 Bake for 40–45
    minutes, or until set
and golden brown.

TUNA MORNAY

Preparation: **10 minutes**
Cooking time: **5 minutes**
SERVES **2**

15 g butter
2 teaspoons plain
    flour
1/2 cup milk
1/4 cup grated cheese
185 g canned tuna
1 tablespoon chopped
    parsley, optional

1 Melt the butter in a
    small pan. Add the
flour and cook, stirring
constantly, over low
heat for 1 minute.

2 Gradually add the
    milk, stirring the
mixture until smooth
between each addition.
When all the milk has
been added, keep
stirring until the
mixture has boiled and
thickened. Cook for
1 minute longer.

3 Remove from the
    heat and stir in the
cheese until melted.
Drain the tuna and
flake with a fork. Stir
into the sauce with the
parsley. Serve warm,
with bread.

FISH PATTIES

Preparation: **15 minutes**
Cooking time: **15 minutes**
MAKES **4**

1 small fish fillet
1 potato, cooked and
    mashed
1/4 cup grated carrot
1/4 cup grated zucchini
1/4 cup grated Cheddar
    cheese
1/4 cup plain flour
olive oil

1 Steam, poach or
    microwave the fish
and break into flakes,
checking carefully for
bones or skin. Mix
together with the
potato, carrot, zucchini
and cheese.

2 Shape into small
    patties or fingers and
dust with flour. Lightly
brush a non-stick pan
with olive oil and cook
the patties slowly until
golden brown. Turn
once during cooking.

3 Drain well on paper
    towels and serve
with wedges of tomato.

From top: *Savoury Flan; Tuna Mornay; Fish Patties*

VEGIE PUFFS

Preparation: **15 minutes**
Cooking time: **15 minutes**
MAKES 24

1 small potato, finely
    chopped
1 small carrot, finely
    chopped
1 small zucchini,
    chopped
1 stalk celery, chopped
1/4 cup chopped
    pumpkin
1/4 cup chopped
    broccoli
1/4 cup chopped
    cauliflower
2 cups grated cheese
2 sheets puff pastry,
    halved
milk, for coating

1 Put the potato,
carrot, zucchini,
celery, pumpkin,
broccoli and
cauliflower in a small
saucepan and add
enough water to cover
them. Bring to the boil,
then reduce the heat
and simmer for
3 minutes. Drain well
and transfer to a bowl
to cool. Add the cheese
to the vegetables and
mix well.

2 Preheat the oven to
220°C. Put the four
pieces of pastry out on
a board, divide the
mixture in four and
spread it along the long
side of each piece.

3 Roll up the pastry to
form sausage shapes,
brush the edge with a
little milk and press to
seal. Place the rolls,
seam side down, on a
lightly greased baking
tray. Make a few small
slits along the rolls.

4 Lightly brush the
rolls with milk to
glaze and then bake for
10 minutes, or until
crisp and golden. Cut
each roll into 6 even-
sized pieces using a
sharp knife.

MUFFIN PIZZAS

Preparation: **10 minutes**
Cooking time: **5 minutes**
SERVES 2

1 English muffin,
    halved
1 tablespoon tomato
    sauce
1/4 cup chopped ham
1/4 cup sliced pineapple
1/2 cup grated
    mozzarella cheese

1 Spread each muffin
half with tomato
sauce. Top with ham
and pineapple and
sprinkle with cheese.

2 Grill until the
cheese melts. Serve
with a small salad.

OMELETTE

Preparation: **5 minutes**
Cooking time: **5 minutes**
SERVES 1

1 egg
1 tablespoon milk
1 teaspoon butter
fillings such as cottage
    cheese, leftover
    vegetables, chopped
    cooked bacon,
    chopped tomato,
    sliced mushrooms or
    grated cheese

1 Whisk together the
egg and milk. Melt
the butter in a small
frying pan and add the
egg mixture, swirling to
cover the pan.

2 When the omelette
is almost set sprinkle
the filling over it. Fold
in half to enclose the
filling. Cook 1 minute
more. Slide onto a
plate and allow to cool.

From top: *Muffin Pizzas; Vegie Puffs; Omelette* ▶

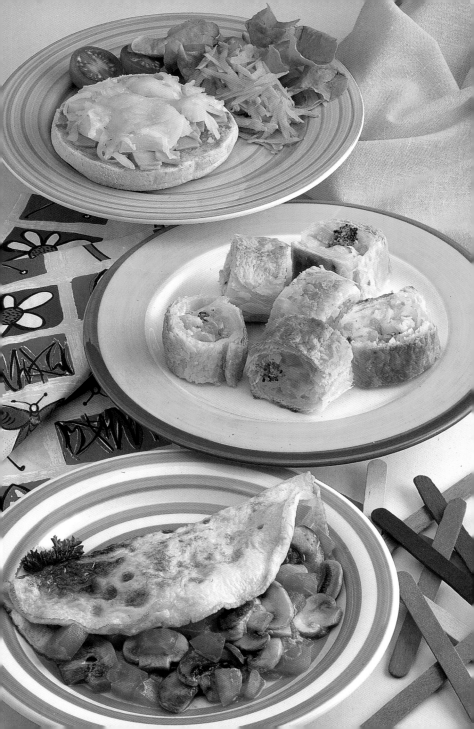

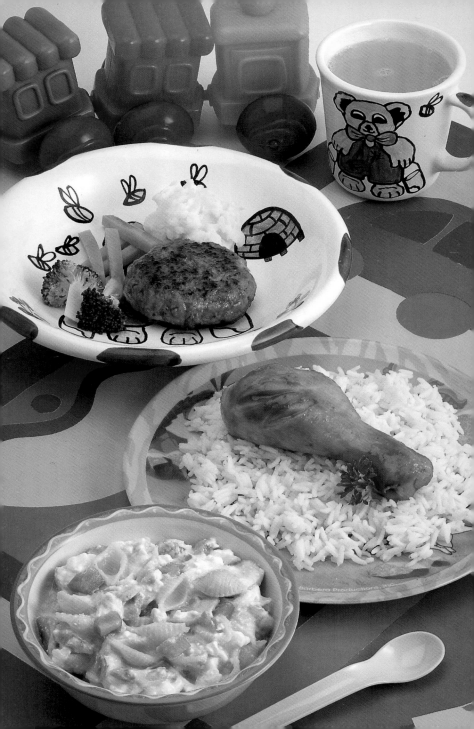

SAVOURY SHELLS

Preparation: **10 minutes**
Cooking time: **10 minutes**
SERVES 1

15 g butter
$^1/_4$ cup chopped
    mushrooms
2 teaspoons plain flour
$^1/_2$ cup milk
$^1/_4$ cup cottage cheese
$^1/_4$ cup grated mild
    Cheddar cheese
1 small tomato, peeled,
    seeded and chopped
$^1/_2$ cup cooked pasta
    shells

1 Melt the butter in a small saucepan and sauté the mushrooms until tender.

2 Stir in the flour and cook for 1 minute. Remove from the heat and gradually blend in the milk, stirring all the time until smooth.

3 Return to the heat. Cook, stirring continuously, until the sauce boils and thickens. Reduce the heat and simmer for 3 minutes.

4 Blend in the cheeses and tomato then gently mix through the pasta shells and serve.

APRICOT DRUMS

Preparation: **35 minutes**
Cooking time: **30 minutes**
SERVES 4

4 chicken drumsticks
$^1/_4$ cup apricot nectar
1 tablespoon soy sauce
2 teaspoons tomato
    sauce
1 teaspoon lemon juice

1 Make a few slashes in each chicken drumstick, using a sharp knife. (For younger toddlers, remove the skin.) Put the drumsticks in a shallow ovenproof dish.

2 Pour over the combined nectar, sauces, lemon juice. Set aside to marinate for about 30 minutes, basting occasionally.

3 Preheat the oven to 180°C and bake, with the marinade, for 30 minutes or until tender, turning once. Serve with rice. Remove the chicken from the bone for younger toddlers. Any extra cooked chicken can be covered and refrigerated for up to one day.

MINI MEAT PATTIES

Preparation: **10 minutes**
Cooking time: **20 minutes**
MAKES 8

500 g lean minced
    steak
1 onion, grated
1 potato, grated
1 carrot, grated
1 egg, beaten
$^1/_4$ cup sultanas
$^1/_4$ cup fresh
    breadcrumbs
2 tablespoons tomato
    sauce
olive oil

1 Mix together all the ingredients and shape into 8 even-sized, flat patties. (If you don't want to cook all the patties, wrap them individually in plastic wrap and freeze for up to 6 months.)

2 Heat a little oil in a frying pan. Cook the patties, in batches if necessary, over medium heat for about 5 minutes each side. Serve with steamed or raw vegetables and mashed potatoes.

From top: *Mini Meat Patties; Apricot Drums; Savoury Shells*

CREAMED RICE

Preparation: **5 minutes**
Cooking time: **25 minutes**
SERVES 4

30 g butter
1 cup short-grain rice
1/4 teaspoon ground
  cinnamon
21/2 cups milk
1/4 cup sugar
1/4 cup sultanas,
  optional

1 Melt the butter in a
  pan and sauté the
rice and cinnamon for
1 minute.

2 Stir in the milk and
  sugar and bring to
the boil. Reduce the
heat and simmer,
stirring occasionally, for
20 minutes, or until the
rice is tender.

3 Blend in the
  sultanas (for older
toddlers). Serve with
fresh fruit.

BAKED CUSTARD

Preparation: **5 minutes**
Cooking time: **20 minutes**
SERVES 2

11/2 cups milk
2 eggs
1 tablespoon sugar
few drops vanilla
  essence
ground nutmeg

1 Preheat the oven to
  180°C. Whisk
together the milk, eggs,
sugar and vanilla
essence. Pour into
2 ramekins or a small
ovenproof dish and
sprinkle with a little
ground nutmeg.

2 Stand the ramekins
  or casserole dish in
an oven tray. Fill the
tray with warm water
to come halfway up the
side of the dish.

3 Bake for about
  15–20 minutes
(35–40 minutes for the
larger dish). When
cooked, the point of a
knife inserted into the
centre of the custard
will come out clean
and dry. Remove the
dish from the water and
allow to cool.

FRUIT KEBABS WITH HONEY AND YOGHURT

Preparation: **15 minutes**
Cooking time: **Nil**
MAKES 4

8 strawberries, hulled
1 banana, chopped
1 kiwi fruit, peeled
  and chopped
1/2 small pineapple,
  peeled and chopped
1/4 rockmelon, seeded
  and chopped
200 g natural yoghurt
2 tablespoons honey

1 Thread pieces of
  fruit alternately onto
4 paddlepop sticks.

2 Blend together the
  yoghurt and honey
and serve as a dipping
sauce for the fruit.

Note: Always toss
banana (or apple and
pear) in lemon juice if
leaving cut for any
length of time or else
it will discolour.

From top: *Creamed Rice; Baked Custard;*
Fruit Kebabs with Honey and Yoghurt ▶

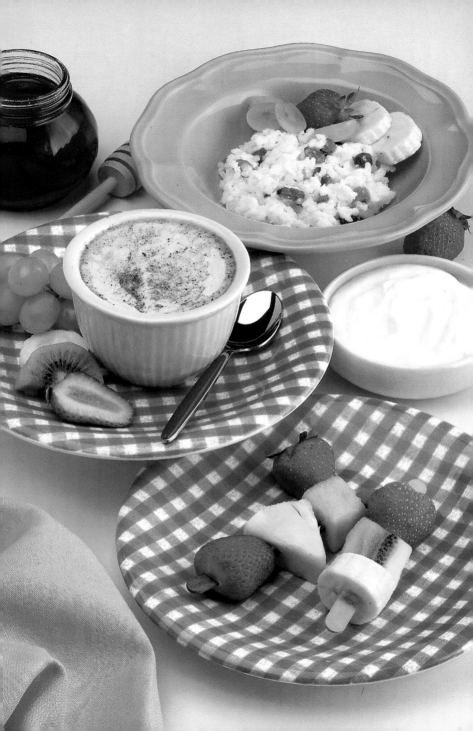

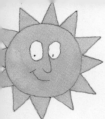

kitchen

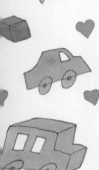

Meal times are usually very busy times in many homes, so for most of us the aim is to prepare foods that the whole family, including baby, will enjoy. This need not be hard work, but does require a little planning and thought. If you have a freezer, microwave and blender, these can all be put to good use.

■ There are not many foods that cannot be frozen—and those that can't should be prepared in smaller quantities and stored in the refrigerator. Always make a little extra so that you have left-overs for tomorrow's dinner or to freeze for a 'meal in a hurry'.

■ Freeze single serves of purées in an ice cube tray or by simply dropping spoonfuls onto a clean tray. Seal in a plastic bag, freeze until firm and then put in labelled and dated plastic bags to reduce the amount of freezer space used. Seal well and remove single cubes as required. Never leave food cubes out of the freezer for any length of time until you are ready to use them.

■ For babies, fish can be frozen for up to 1 month, meat for up to 3 months, offal for up to 1 month, fruit and vegetables for up to 3 months and soups and baked goods for up to 6 months.

■ Plan meals on a weekly basis and buy fruit, vegetables and meat in larger quantities. Cook them for puréeing, mashing or chopping at one time and then freeze. Remember to keep two days supply in the refrigerator and think ahead, transferring frozen portions to the refrigerator when supplies are running low.

■ Great care must be taken when using the microwave oven to heat food for your baby. Remember that food continues to cook for several seconds after the heating time is complete and is therefore very hot. Always test before serving.

hints

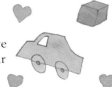

■ Always refer to the manufacturer's manual for microwave defrosting programmes. Loosen all covers and wraps and remove any metal ties before defrosting. For even defrosting, turn or stir food occasionally.

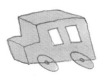

■ To reheat frozen baby foods, use a microwave or put in a dish over a saucepan of simmering water. The microwave is also ideal for cooking fruit and vegetables for puréeing.

■ Always mix food thoroughly during and after heating, as the outside could be very hot while the inside is still cold. Leave it to stand for several minutes before serving.

■ Make your own teething rusks by placing 6 thick chunks of bread in the microwave. Cook on High (100%) power for 1 minute. Allow to stand for 1 minute. If the rusks need further cooking to dry out thoroughly (this will depend on the type of bread used), use short, 30-second bursts.

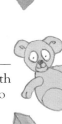

■ Cook baby portions of rice or pasta in the microwave oven—$1/2$ cup rice or pasta in a large microwave-safe casserole dish with 1 cup water. Cook on High (100%) power, uncovered, for 10 to 12 minutes.

■ When preparing food for the whole family, set aside your baby's serving before adding any spices or strong flavourings.

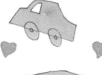

■ As babies like soft food, it is tempting to overcook fruit and vegetables. However, try not to do this and, if possible, use any cooking liquid for puréeing to help retain the nutrients.

■ Keep a supply of fruit (fresh and dried), teething biscuits, cheese, grated vegetables for snacks for older babies and toddlers.

PICNIC FOOD

Taking your toddler to the park or the beach? Make it a real day out with a portable packed lunch.

CHEESY PIZZA

Preparation: **15 minutes**
Cooking time: **20 minutes**
MAKES **12 WEDGES**

2 cups self-raising
   flour
30 g butter, chopped
1/2 cup milk
1/2 cup water

Topping:
1 cup grated cheese
1 tomato, finely
   chopped
1/4 cup ricotta cheese
1/4 cup chopped ham
1 tablespoon chopped
   parsley

1 Preheat the oven to 220°C. Sift the flour into a bowl and use your fingertips to rub in the butter until it looks like breadcrumbs. Make a well in the centre and pour in the combined milk and water.

2 Mix quickly into a soft dough and turn onto a lightly floured surface. Knead lightly. Press or roll out to a circle 1 cm thick.

3 Put the pizza base on an oiled oven tray. Mix together all the topping ingredients and spoon over the pastry, leaving a border round the edge.

4 Bake for 20 minutes. Cut into slices and serve with salad.

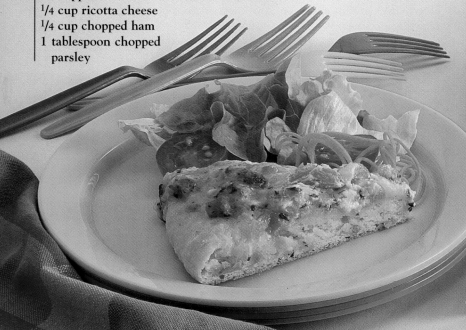

MINI QUICHE LORRAINES

Preparation: **10 minutes**
Cooking time: **25 minutes**
MAKES 12

2 sheets frozen ready-
  rolled shortcrust
  pastry, thawed
1 tomato, chopped
1/2 cup grated tasty
  cheese
1/4 cup chopped ham
  or bacon
1 spring onion, finely
  chopped
1/2 cup milk
1 egg

1 Preheat the oven to 180°C. Cut the pastry into 12 rounds using a 7.5 cm cutter. Line 12 shallow patty tins with the pastry. Cut pieces of greaseproof paper to cover each pastry shell. Fill with uncooked rice, chickpeas or baking beans and bake blind for 5 minutes. Remove the paper and rice, peas or beans and bake for a further 2 minutes. Cool before filling.

2 Mix together the tomato, cheese, ham and spring onion and spoon into the tins.

3 Whisk together the milk and egg. Pour enough into each tin to cover the filling.

4 Bake in the oven for 15–20 minutes, or until the filling is set and golden.

5 Transfer to a wire rack to cool. Store in the refrigerator in an airtight container for up to two days.

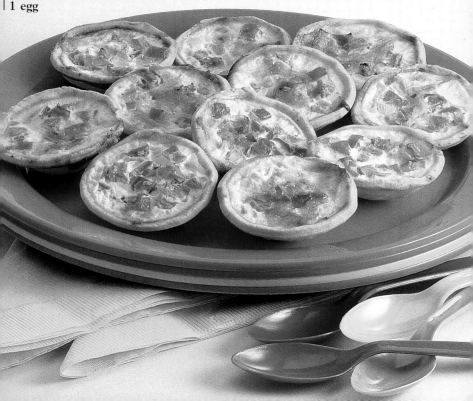

SHORTBREADS

Preparation: **15 minutes**
Cooking time: **30 minutes**
MAKES 16 PIECES

2 cups plain flour
2 tablespoons rice
   flour
1/2 cup caster sugar
250 g butter,
   chopped

1 Preheat the oven
to 160°C. Sift the
flours together into a
large bowl and mix in
the sugar. Rub in the
butter using your
fingertips and press the
mixture together.

2 Turn out onto a
lightly floured
surface and knead
gently. Press out into a
round about 1 cm
thick and cut out
with shaped cutters.
Put onto greased
baking trays.

3 Bake for 25–30
minutes, or until
golden brown.

4 Leave to cool on the
trays for 5 minutes
and then transfer to a
wire rack to cool
completely. Store in an
airtight container.

From top: *Orange Cake;
Scones; Shortbreads*

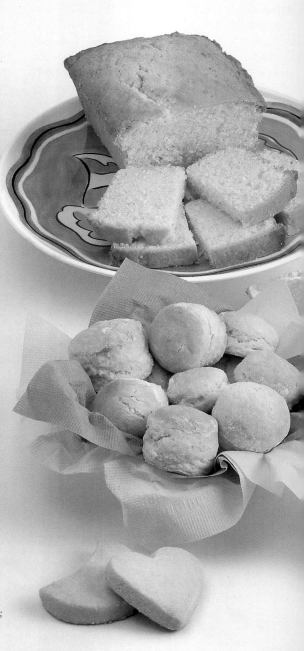

SCONES

Preparation: **10 minutes**
Cooking time: **12 minutes**
MAKES ABOUT **12**

**2 cups self-raising
  flour
30 g butter, chopped
1/2 cup milk
1/2 cup water**

1 Preheat the oven to
220°C. Sift the flour
into a large bowl and
rub in the butter using
your fingertips.

2 Make a well in the
centre of the flour.
Pour in the combined
milk and water, saving
1 teaspoonful to glaze.
Mix quickly to a soft
dough with a knife.

3 Turn onto a lightly
floured board and
knead lightly. Press or
roll out to form a round
about 2 cm thick.

4 Cut into rounds or
wedges and put
close together on a
greased scone tray.
Glaze with the reserved
milk and water mix.

5 Bake for 10–12
minutes, or until the
scones sound hollow
when tapped. Cool on
a wire rack.

ORANGE CAKE

Preparation: **10 minutes**
Cooking time: **45 minutes**
MAKES **1** CAKE

**125 g butter
1/2 cup caster sugar
2 eggs
1 teaspoon vanilla
  essence
grated rind of 1 orange
2 cups self-raising
  flour, sifted
1/4 cup orange juice
1/4 cup milk**

1 Preheat the oven to
180°C. Beat the
butter and sugar
together until light
and fluffy.

2 Add the eggs one at
a time, beating well.
Beat in the vanilla
essence and rind.

3 Fold the flour into
the mixture
alternately with the
combined juice and
milk, beginning and
ending with the flour.

4 Spoon the mixture
into a greased and
floured 10 x 20 cm loaf
tin and bake for
40–45 minutes. Leave
to cool in the tin for a
few minutes, then turn
out onto a wire rack.

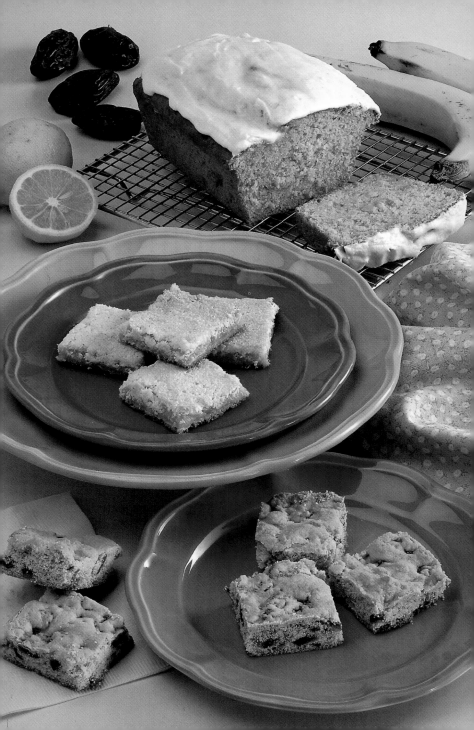

BANANA CAKE

Preparation: **10 minutes**
Cooking time: **45 minutes**
MAKES 1 LOAF

125 g butter
1/2 cup brown sugar
2 eggs
1 cup mashed banana
  (about 3 ripe
  bananas)
1/2 cup sour cream
2 cups self-raising
  flour, sifted

Icing:
1 1/2 cups icing sugar,
  sifted
15 g soft butter
1 teaspoon grated
  lemon rind
1–2 tablespoons lemon
  juice

1 Preheat the oven to
180°C. Cream the
butter and sugar
together until fluffy.
Add the eggs one at a
time, beating well. Stir
in the mashed banana
and sour cream.

2 Lightly fold in the
flour. Spoon the
mixture into a greased
and lined 23 x 13 cm
loaf tin.

3 Bake for 40–45
minutes, or until a
skewer inserted into
the centre comes out
clean. Turn onto a wire
rack to cool.

4 Mix together all the
icing ingredients
until smooth, then
spread over the cooled
cake. If necessary, the
cake can be wrapped in
freezer wrap and frozen.

DATE SQUARES

Preparation: **10 minutes**
Cooking time: **25 minutes**
MAKES ABOUT 24

90 g butter
3/4 cup brown sugar
1 egg
1 1/2 cups self-raising
flour, sifted
1 cup chopped dates

1 Preheat the oven to
180°C. Cream
together the butter and
sugar until well
combined. Add the
egg and beat well.

2 Gently fold in the
flour, followed by
the dates. Press gently
into a greased shallow
18 x 28 cm tin.

3 Bake for 20–25
minutes, or until
lightly golden brown.
Cut into squares.

MERINGUE SLICE

Preparation: **15 minutes**
Cooking time: **30 minutes**
MAKES ABOUT 24

125 g butter
1 cup caster sugar
2 eggs, separated
1 cup self-raising
  flour, sifted
1 cup desiccated
  coconut

1 Preheat the oven to
180°C. Cream the
butter and half the
sugar together until
light and fluffy. Add
the egg yolks and beat.

2 Fold in the flour.
Flour your fingertips
and press the dough
into the base of a
greased 18 x 28 cm tin.

3 Beat the egg whites
into stiff peaks.
Gradually beat in the
rest of the sugar until
thick and glossy. Fold
in the coconut.

4 Spread the meringue
over the pastry base.
Bake for 25–30
minutes, or until a
skewer comes out clean
when inserted into the
centre. Cool, then cut
into squares. Store in
an airtight container.

From top: *Banana Cake; Meringue Slice; Date Squares*

TODDLER DINNERS

Dinner times become easier and much more fun when your toddler is able to join the family for meals.

CREAMY CHICKEN AND CORN SOUP

Preparation: **5 minutes**
Cooking time: **25 minutes**
MAKES ABOUT 1 LITRE

1 litre chicken stock
1 cup finely chopped cooked chicken
130 g creamed corn
1/4 cup small pasta
1 tablespoon chopped parsley

1 Place the stock, chicken, corn and pasta in a pan. Bring to the boil and then reduce the heat and simmer for 15–20 minutes, or until the pasta is very tender.

2 Stir in the parsley and allow to cool. Process until smooth in a food processor or blender. Reheat or refrigerate in an airtight container for up to 5 days or freeze in portion sizes.

MINESTRONE

Preparation: **15 minutes**
Cooking time: **1½ hours**
MAKES 3½ LITRES

2 tablespoons olive oil
1 onion, chopped
1 rasher rindless bacon, finely chopped
3 carrots, chopped
3 zucchini, sliced
2 stalks, celery, sliced
2 potatoes, peeled and chopped
125 g green beans, trimmed and sliced
425 g can tomatoes
300 g can 4-bean mix, drained and rinsed
10 cups (2½ litres) water
1/3 cup small pasta
grated Parmesan cheese
chopped parsley

1 Heat the oil in a large saucepan and sauté the onion and bacon until the onion is tender. Add the carrot, zucchini, celery, potatoes, beans, tomatoes and bean mix and cook, stirring, for 1 minute.

2 Add the water to the pan and season to taste with pepper and herbs of your choice. Bring to the boil and then reduce the heat and simmer, covered, for 1 hour.

3 Stir in the pasta and simmer for a further 15 minutes, or until tender. Sprinkle the Minestrone with cheese and parsley and serve with crusty bread.

Croutons: Cut the crusts from 4 slices of bread and cut the bread into cubes. Heat 30 g butter and 1 tablespoon oil in a small frying pan. Add the bread in batches and fry, turning, until crisp and golden. Drain on paper towels. Store in an airtight container.

From top: *Creamy Chicken and Corn Soup; Minestrone* ▶

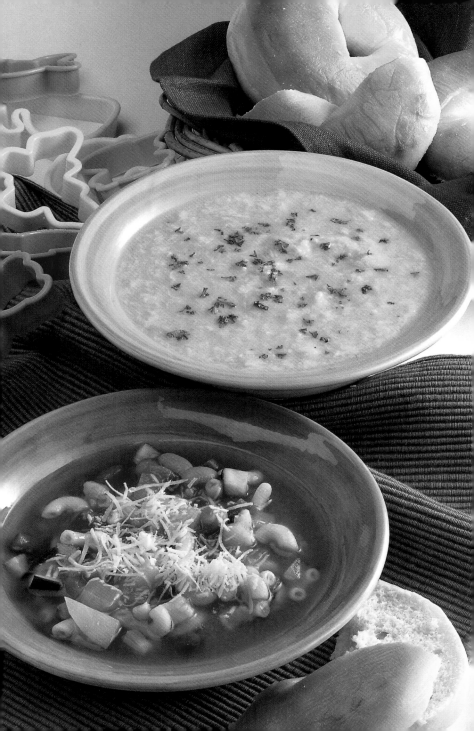

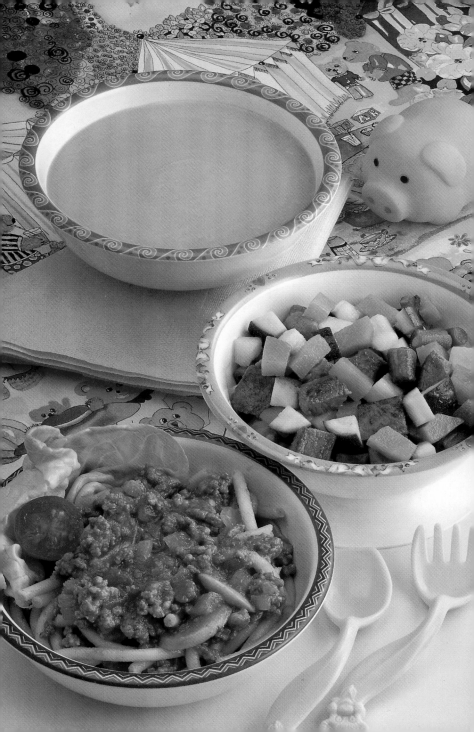

SIMPLE BOLOGNESE

Preparation: **10 minutes**
Cooking time: **30 minutes**
SERVES 8

2 tablespoons olive oil
1 onion, finely
  chopped
1 clove garlic, crushed
500 g minced steak
1/4 cup chopped
  mushrooms
2 tablespoons tomato
  paste
425 g can tomatoes,
  chopped
1/2 cup beef stock
  or water
1 tablespoon chopped
  parsley
seasoning, to taste
cooked pasta of choice

1 Heat the oil in a
  heavy-based pan and
sauté the onion and
garlic until tender. Add
the mince and brown
well, breaking up with
a spoon as it cooks.

2 Add the mushrooms
  and cook for 1
minute. Blend in the
tomato paste.

3 Stir in the tomatoes,
  stock, parsley and
seasoning. Bring to the
boil and then reduce

the heat and simmer,
stirring occasionally,
for 20 minutes.

4 Toss the sauce
  through hot,
drained pasta. Sprinkle
with grated Parmesan
or Cheddar, if liked,
and serve with salad.

Note: If you can't
find chopped tinned
tomatoes, buy whole
tinned tomatoes and
chop them in the tin
with a pair of scissors
or sharp knife.

CARROT AND POTATO SOUP

Preparation: **10 minutes**
Cooking time: **35 minutes**
SERVES 4

15 g butter or 1
  tablespoon olive oil
3 carrots, chopped
1 potato, peeled and
  chopped
1 litre chicken or
  vegetable stock
milk

1 Melt the butter or
  oil in a medium-
sized saucepan. Add the
carrot and potato and
cook over low heat for
3 minutes.

2 Pour in the stock
  and bring to the
boil. Reduce the heat
and simmer for 25–30
minutes, or until the
vegetables are very
tender. Allow to cool.

3 Process the soup in
  a food processor or
blender until smooth.
Refrigerate in an
airtight container for
up to five days or freeze
in serving portions.
Reheat with a little
milk to taste.

TODDLER COMBO

Preparation: **10 minutes**
Cooking time: **25 minutes**
SERVES 2

1 potato, peeled and
  chopped
1 carrot, chopped
1 zucchini, chopped
1/2 cup chopped sweet
  potato
1/4 cup chopped green
  beans
1/2 cup chopped
  cooked meat

1 Steam, boil or
  microwave the
vegetables until tender
and then mix with the
meat to serve.

◀ **From top:** *Carrot and Potato Soup;*
Toddler Combo; Simple Bolognese

MACARONI CHEESE

Preparation: **5 minutes**
Cooking time: **10 minutes**
SERVES 4

30 g butter
1 tablespoon plain
   flour
1 cup milk
seasoning, to taste
1/2 cup grated cheese
2 cups cooked
   macaroni

1 Melt the butter in a small saucepan. Blend in the flour and cook for 1 minute.

2 Remove from the heat and gradually blend in the milk. Return to the heat and cook, stirring, until the sauce boils and thickens.

3 Reduce the heat and simmer for 3 minutes. Season and stir in the cheese. Mix the macaroni through the sauce and serve with tomato wedges.

Note: The mixture can be put into ramekins and topped with a little grated cheese and dry breadcrumbs, then baked in a 180°C oven for 5–10 minutes or until golden. Allow the ramekins to cool before serving.

APRICOT CHICKEN

Preparation: **10 minutes**
Cooking time: **50 minutes**
SERVES 4–6

500 g chicken thigh
   fillets, chopped, skin
   removed
125 g mushrooms,
   sliced
1 onion, thinly sliced
45 g packet chicken
   noodle soup
420 g canned apricots
   in their own juice
125 g green beans or
   snow peas, trimmed

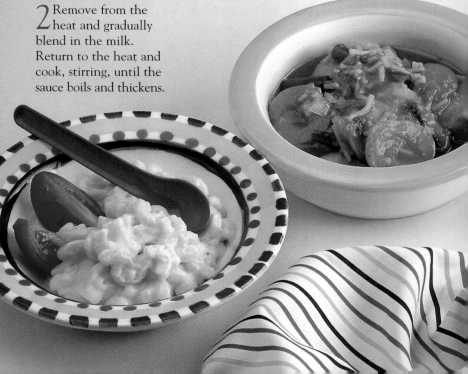

PASTA BAKE

Preparation: **10 minutes**
Cooking time: **1 hour**
SERVES 4–6

250 g pasta, cooked
  and drained
125 g ricotta cheese
3 eggs
1 tablespoon olive oil
1 onion, chopped
500 g minced steak,
  lamb, pork or
  chicken
425 g can tomatoes,
  chopped
1/2 cup water
2 tablespoons tomato
  paste
300 ml cream
1 1/2 cups grated cheese
1/2 cup fresh
  breadcrumbs

1 Combine the pasta with the ricotta and 1 egg. Press into a greased casserole dish.

2 Heat the oil in a pan and cook the onion until tender. Add the mince and brown well.

3 Stir in the tomatoes, water and tomato paste. Simmer, uncovered, for 15–20 minutes, or until the sauce begins to thicken, and then spoon over the pasta.

4 Whisk together the cream, remaining eggs and 1 cup cheese and pour over the meat mixture. Combine the remaining cheese and the breadcrumbs and sprinkle over the top.

5 Bake at 180°C for 35–40 minutes, or until golden.

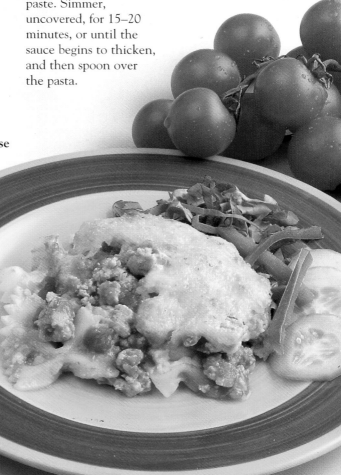

FAMILY CASSEROLE

Preparation: **10 minutes**
Cooking time: **3 hours**
SERVES **4–6**

75 g butter
2 tablespoons oil
1 kg round steak, cut
  into 2 cm cubes
6 small onions
4 potatoes, peeled
  and halved
3 carrots, halved
2 parsnips, chopped
1/3 cup plain flour
5 cups beef stock
1/4 cup tomato paste
1 teaspoon
  Worcestershire
  sauce
chopped parsley

1 Heat 15 g butter with the oil in a large pan. Add the meat in batches and brown well on all sides. Remove to a plate.

2 Add the onions, potatoes, carrots and parsnips to the pan and cook until golden. Remove to the plate and cover with foil.

3 Add the remaining butter to the pan and stir in the flour. Cook, stirring, until golden brown and then remove from the heat.

4 Gradually blend in the stock, tomato paste, sauce, salt and pepper and return to the heat. Cook, stirring continuously, until the sauce boils and thickens.

5 Return the meat to the pan, stirring to coat it in sauce. Bring to the boil and then reduce the heat and simmer, covered, for 1 1/2–2 hours.

6 Add the reserved vegetables. Simmer for 30 minutes, or until the vegetables are tender. Transfer the meat and vegetables to a serving plate and keep warm.

7 Bring the sauce to the boil and then reduce the heat and simmer, uncovered, until slightly thickened. Sprinkle the meat and vegetables with parsley and serve with sauce.

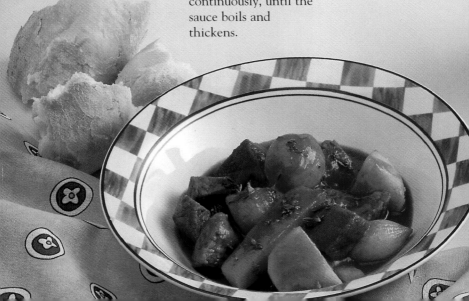

PASTA AND VEGETABLE GRATIN

Preparation: **10 minutes**
Cooking time: **30 minutes**
SERVES 2

1 cup chopped mixed
   vegetables
2 cups cooked pasta
30 g butter
1 tablespoon plain
   flour
1 cup milk
1/4 cup grated cheese
1 tablespoon dried
   breadcrumbs

1 Preheat the oven to 180°C. Steam, boil or microwave the vegetables in a little water, until tender. Put in a greased casserole dish with the pasta and stir to combine.

2 Melt the butter in a small pan. Blend in the flour and cook, stirring, for 1 minute.

3 Gradually blend in the milk until smooth. Cook, stirring, until the sauce boils and thickens. Simmer for 3 minutes. Pour over the vegetables.

4 Mix together the cheese and breadcrumbs and sprinkle over the top. Bake for 15 minutes.

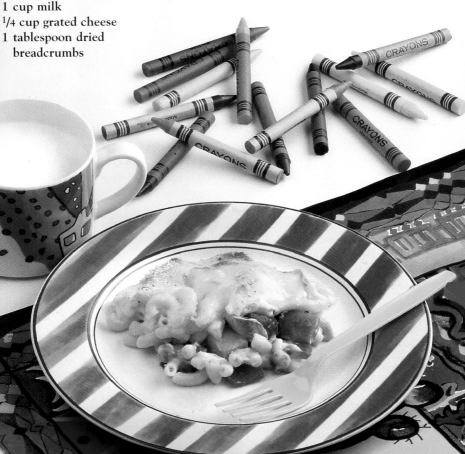

PEAR CRUMBLE

Preparation: **5 minutes**
Cooking time: **40 minutes**
SERVES **4–6**

....

4 pears, peeled, cored
    and sliced
1 tablespoon caster
    sugar
2 cups plain or
    wholemeal plain
    flour, sifted
125 g butter, chopped
1/2 cup brown sugar

1 Preheat the oven to
    190°C. Place the
fruit in the base of a
greased ovenproof dish
and sprinkle with sugar.
2 Put the flour in a
    bowl. Rub in the
butter with your
fingertips until the
mixture is crumbly. Stir
in the brown sugar.
3 Sprinkle the
    crumble topping
over the fruit. Bake for
35–40 minutes, or until
golden. Serve warm
with custard.

Note: Use apples
and rhubarb or other
fruit, or berries for
older toddlers. Try
adding a tablespoon
of coconut to the
crumble topping.

VANILLA ICE CREAM

Preparation: **5 minutes**
Cooking time: **15 minutes**
SERVES **4**

....

1 cup milk
1 cup cream
1 teaspoon vanilla
    essence
2 eggs
2 egg yolks
1/2 cup caster sugar

1 Put the milk and
    cream in a small
saucepan. Bring to the
boil and then remove
from the heat. Stir in
the vanilla essence.
2 Whisk the eggs, egg
    yolks and sugar
together in a heat-
resistant bowl. Whisk
in the milk mixture.
3 Place the bowl over
    a saucepan of gently
simmering water and
whisk until the mixture
thickens and coats the
back of a metal spoon.
4 Pour the custard
    into a metal tray
and freeze until it is
semi-solid.
5 Beat the mixture
    thoroughly, either
in a food processor or
by hand, to remove the

ice crystals. Return to
the tray, cover with foil
and freeze until firm.
Serve with fruit, wafers,
toppings or in a cone.

Note: To make a
fruity ice cream, just
stir in 2 cups chopped
or puréed fruit after
processing the ice
cream and then freeze
until firm.

TRIFLE MAGIC

Preparation: **15 minutes**
Cooking time: **Nil**
SERVES **4**

....

1 ready-made swiss
    roll, sliced
85 g packet jelly, set
    in a tray
2 cups chopped fruit
1 cup prepared custard

1 Arrange the cake in
    the bases of small
serving dishes. Chop
the jelly roughly, mix
with the fruit and
spoon over the cake.
2 Pour over the
    custard and serve
with ice cream.

From top: *Vanilla Ice Cream;*
Trifle Magic; Pear Crumble

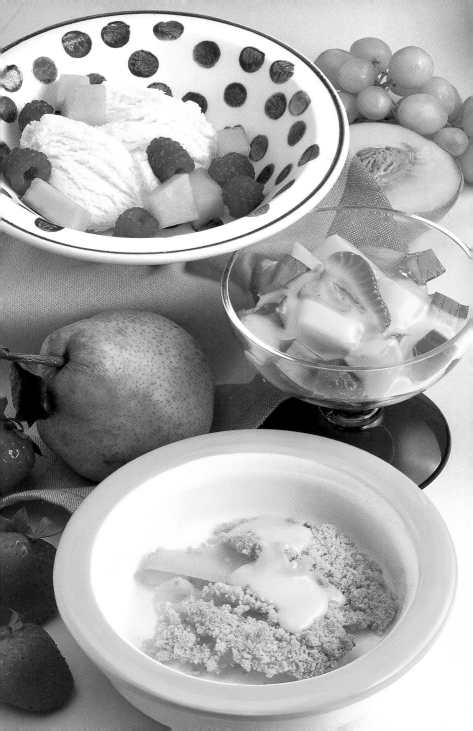

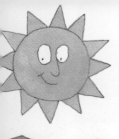

fussy

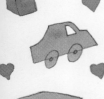

Without warning your child may begin to refuse once-loved food. This is not necessarily a criticism of your culinary skills but just as likely to be his first assertion of individual choice. Don't panic—remember that he will always eat when he is hungry. Run through the following checklist to see if there is anything you can do to help.

■ Make sure meal times are happy and relaxed. If meal times become associated with anger they will become more stressful for both of you, with your baby even less inclined to eat. Don't insist that your child finishes everything. If he refuses food do not offer substitutes but wait until the next meal.

■ Are you still puréeing food when your older baby has progressed beyond that? Or overestimating his ability to chew by offering large solid pieces?

■ Children are creatures of habit. Keep meals to regular times and give him his own chair and utensils. If he seems unsettled and won't eat, consider if there have been any recent changes that have threatened his security.

■ Try disguising nutritious food your child has rejected by mixing it in with an old favourite such as mashed potatoes.

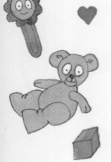

■ Serve small portions, giving seconds if they are asked for. Three small meals and two snacks daily suit most children better than three dauntingly large meals. Don't put too much on the plate and always try to make it look attractive.

■ Any child who is upset, tired, teething or not feeling well is unlikely to want to eat.

eaters

■ Remember that children have growth spurts. A baby grows a proportionately large amount in his first year but you will find that a 5-year old often only eats as much as a 1-year old.

■ Has your child been given snacks throughout the day? Too much milk or fruit juice will take the edge off any appetite. Two cups of orange juice are equivalent to four oranges.

■ Encourage his appetite through fresh air, exercise and sleep—perhaps he has been less active than usual and isn't as hungry.

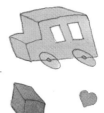

■ Genuine dislikes are often formed early—if certain foods are always left on the plate or spat out, this may be a sign to avoid these for a while. Always try them again at a later date.

■ To encourage good eating habits, don't always serve a sweet dessert after a savoury. Stick to one-course meals with desserts occasionally. Don't bribe children with sweet foods—this only makes them seem more special.

■ Most children are hungriest mid-afternoon. Don't let him fill up on cakes, biscuits and lollies then but, if it is practical, serve the main meal of the day, with a snack at dinner time.

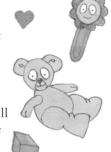

■ Encourage your toddler to take an interest in food by helping with the preparation. Talk about the food as you cook and let him add herbs and spices then taste for flavour. Offer a choice of food to make him feel grown-up.

■ For older toddlers, try a little subtle deception. Put home-made sandwiches into a bag to pretend they've been bought, and custards into well-washed yoghurt cartons.

SNACKS AND NIBBLES

Toddlers lead very busy lives... always rushing about looking for something new to explore. Often children need a quick snack to top up their energy levels. Instead of letting them fill up on sugar and additives, make your own healthy treats.

From top: *Yoghurt Dip; Crunchy Cheese Bites; Bruschetta*

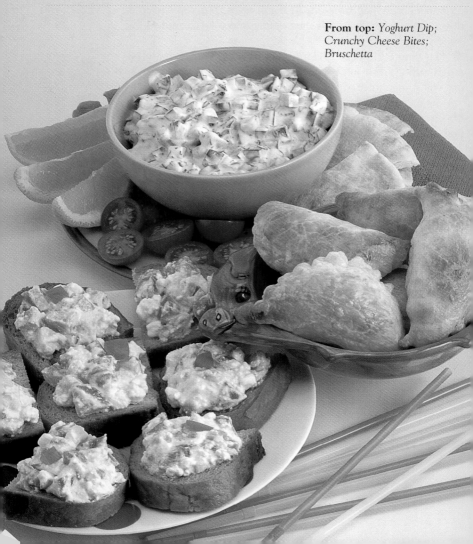

CRUNCHY CHEESE BITES

Preparation: **15 minutes**
Cooking time: **15 minutes**
MAKES ABOUT **20**

2 cups grated cheese
125 g feta cheese, crumbled
1/4 cup ricotta cheese
1/4 cup chopped spring onions
1 small tomato, chopped
1 egg, beaten
pepper, to taste
5 sheets ready-rolled puff pastry
beaten egg and milk, to brush

1 Preheat the oven to 220°C. Combine the cheeses, spring onions, tomato, egg and pepper in a bowl.

2 Cut the pastry into rounds using a 10 cm cutter. Place heaped teaspoons of the mixture onto one half of each round.

3 Fold the pastry over the filling to make semi-circles, brush the edge with a little egg and press the edges together firmly with a fork to seal.

4 Place on a baking tray and brush with a little milk. Bake in the oven for 10–15 minutes, or until puffed and golden. Allow to cool for at least 10 minutes before serving.

BRUSCHETTA

Preparation: **5 minutes**
Cooking time: **10 minutes**
MAKES ABOUT **12 SLICES**

1 Italian loaf, sliced
1/2 cup olive oil
250 g cottage cheese
2 tomatoes, chopped
1 avocado, chopped

1 Preheat the oven to 200°C. Arrange the bread on an oiled baking tray and brush liberally with oil.

2 Bake for 10 minutes, or until golden. Cool and then store the Bruschetta in an airtight container until it is needed.

3 Mix together the cottage cheese, tomatoes and avocado. Spread over the Bruschetta or serve with it as a dip.

YOGHURT DIP

Preparation: **15 minutes**
Cooking time: **Nil**
MAKES **1 CUP**

2 Lebanese cucumbers, seeded and chopped
200 g natural yoghurt, drained
2 cloves garlic, crushed
1 teaspoon lemon juice
1 teaspoon chopped dill
1/2 teaspoon chopped mint

1 Wrap the cucumber in a tea towel and squeeze out the water.

2 Mix the cucumber with the yoghurt, garlic, lemon juice, dill and mint. Serve with small pieces of pitta bread, vegetables such as cucumber or cherry tomatoes, and even sliced fruit.

Note: Don't give young children hard vegetables or fruit, such as carrot or apple, for dipping. Pieces can easily break off and lead to choking. Always grate hard food for young children and toddlers.

PARTY FOOD

There are few events more exciting for toddlers than a party. Ask a friend to help and don't be too ambitious.

CHEESE TWISTS

Preparation: **10 minutes**
Cooking time: **10 minutes**
MAKES ABOUT **30**

2 sheets ready-rolled
   puff pastry
tomato sauce or
   Vegemite
1 cup grated Cheddar
   cheese

1 Preheat the oven to 220°C. Spread one sheet of pastry with tomato sauce or Vegemite and sprinkle with cheese.

2 Put the second piece of pastry on top and press the edges to seal.

3 Cut into 1 cm strips, then cut each strip into three pieces. Twist and put on a lightly greased baking tray.

4 Bake in the oven for about 10 minutes, or until golden and puffed. Cool on a wire rack.

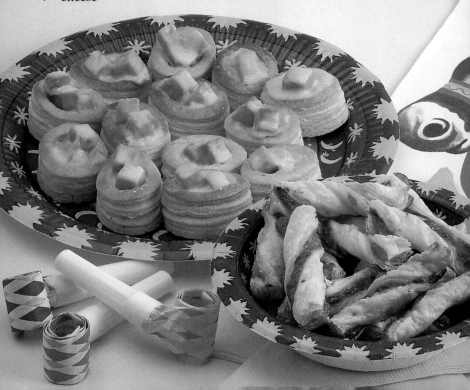

CORNY NESTS

Preparation: **5 minutes**
Cooking time: **15 minutes**
MAKES 24

30 g butter
2 tablespoons plain
 flour
1/2 cup milk
1/2 cup cream
130 g creamed corn
1/2 cup chopped ham
24 small vol-au-vent
 cases

1 Melt the butter in a small saucepan. Add the flour and cook, stirring, for 1 minute.

2 Remove from the heat and gradually blend in the combined milk and cream. Return to the heat and cook, stirring constantly until the sauce boils and thickens. Simmer for 3 minutes.

3 Blend in the corn and ham and spoon into warm vol-au-vent cases (reheated according to the packet directions).

MEATBALLS

Preparation: **10 minutes**
Cooking time: **10 minutes**
MAKES ABOUT 60

500 g sausage mince
500 g minced steak
35 g packet French
 onion soup
1/4 cup tomato sauce
2 tablespoons chopped
 parsley
2 tablespoons oil

1 Mix together the sausage, steak, soup mix, sauce and parsley. Wet your hands to prevent sticking and then mould the mixture into balls.

2 Heat the oil in a frying pan. Add half the meatballs, tossing over medium heat for about 5 minutes, or until cooked through.

3 Drain well on crumpled paper towels and repeat with the remaining balls. Serve warm.

Left to right:
Corny Nests;
Cheese Twists;
Meatballs

BABY ECLAIRS

Preparation: **15 minutes**
Cooking time: **40 minutes**
MAKES ABOUT **24**

75 g butter
1 cup plain flour
4 eggs
125 g dark chocolate, melted
whipped cream

1 Preheat the oven to 200°C. Put the butter in a pan with 1 cup water. Bring to the boil; sift in all the flour.

2 Cook, stirring, until the mixture forms a ball. Transfer to a bowl and cool for 5 minutes.

3 Add the eggs, one at a time, beating well until thick and glossy. Spoon into a piping bag with a plain nozzle and pipe short lengths onto a greased baking tray. Sprinkle with a little water.

4 Bake for 10–15 minutes. Reduce the oven to 180°C and bake for a further 10–15 minutes, or until golden and firm.

5 Pierce the side of each éclair with a skewer to allow steam to escape. Turn off the oven and leave the éclairs inside for about 5 minutes to dry out. Cool on a wire rack.

6 Split the éclairs in half lengthways and remove any uncooked pastry. Spread the tops with chocolate, allow to set, fill with cream and replace the tops.

CHOCOLATE SPONGE

Preparation: **10 minutes**
Cooking time: **20 minutes**
MAKES **1 CAKE**

3 eggs, separated
3/4 cup caster sugar
1 cup self-raising flour, sifted
60 g chocolate, melted
3 tablespoons water

1 Preheat the oven to 180°C. Grease a deep 20 cm round or square cake tin and dust with flour. Beat the egg whites in a clean dry bowl until stiff peaks form. Beat in the sugar until thick and glossy.

2 Beat in the egg yolks. Gently fold in the flour and then the chocolate and water.

3 Pour into the tin and bake for 15–20 minutes, or until the cake springs back when pressed. Cool on a wire rack. Decorate with cream, jam or butter cream or as a party cake (pages 62–63).

BUTTER CREAM

Beat 125 g butter until creamy and gradually add 1 1/2 cups sifted icing sugar. Beat until thick and smooth. Leave plain or colour and flavour with melted chocolate, orange or lemon juice, food colouring etc.

MERINGUES

Preheat the oven to 150°C. Line a baking tray with foil or baking paper. Beat 3 egg whites until stiff. Gradually blend in 1/2 cup caster sugar until thick and glossy. Fold in 1/3 cup caster sugar and spoon or pipe small mounds onto the tray. Bake for 1 to 1 1/2 hours, or until dry. Cool and store in an airtight container.

From top: *Chocolate Sponge topped with cream; Baby Eclairs; Meringues*

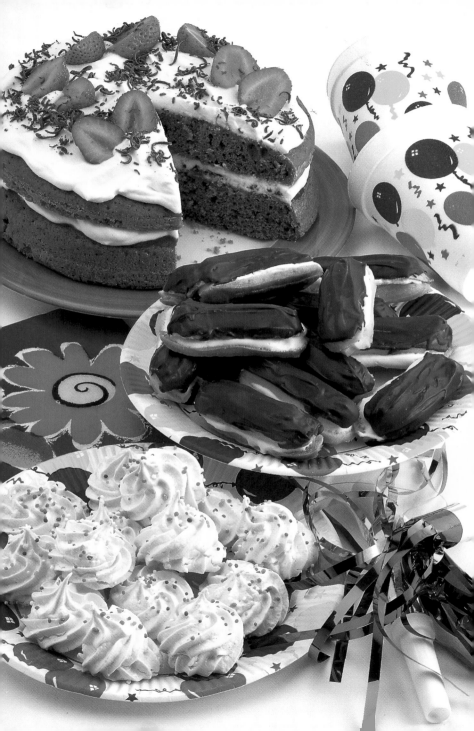

BUNNY CAKE

20 cm square sponge
  cake (page 60)
2 quantities butter
  cream (page 60)
pink food colouring
2 milk arrowroot
  biscuits
2 white chocolate
  melts
2 brown Smarties
2 bright pink musk
  sticks
small liquorice strap
2 white mini
  marshmallows

1 Cut the cake in half.
  Cut one piece in
half again. Put the long
piece and one of the
quarters together to
make a number 1.

2 Cut the remaining
  piece of cake in half
again and place at the
base to make feet. Cut
the ends of the feet to
round them a little.
Leave a small portion
of butter cream white
and tint the rest pink.

3 Stick the pieces of
  cake together with
butter cream. Spread
the rest over the cake
and over the arrowroot
biscuits to make ears as
shown. Decorate the
bunny's face with the
lollies as shown.

Note: Although it is
tempting at parties,
  don't give young
    children hard lollies,
nuts or popcorn—they
can easily lead to
choking. Make sure
toddlers sit quietly,
rather than running
around or playing,
while they eat.

FARMYARD CAKE

20 cm square sponge
  cake (page 60)
1 1/2 quantities butter
  cream (page 60)
1/2 cup desiccated
  coconut, toasted
green and brown food
  colouring
chocolate sticks
Curly Wurly bars
2 rectangular lollies
  for feed bins
shredded coconut
farmyard figures

1 Trim the sides of the
  cake and cover with
butter cream, roughing
up the surface.

2 Put 2 tablespoons of
  the coconut in a
plastic bag with 2–3
drops brown colouring
and shake to combine.
Repeat with the
remaining coconut and
green colouring.

3 Sprinkle the green
  coconut over the
cake and brown
coconut around the
outside edge. Stick the
chocolate sticks in the
corners as fence posts.
Cut the Curly Wurly
bars to fit as fences.
Arrange the feed bins,
animals and gate.

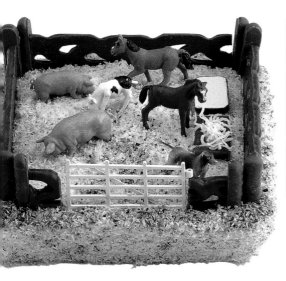

CLOCK CAKE

20 cm round sponge
  cake (page 60)
1 quantity butter
  cream (page 60)
blue food colouring
lots of Smarties
fruit straps, roll-ups or
  other flat lollies
2 different coloured
  jelly snakes
1 freckle lolly

1 Tint the butter
  cream to a bright
blue and cover the
cake. Arrange the
Smarties around
the side.

2 Use a small sharp
  pair of scissors to cut
the numbers from the
flat fruit strap lollies
and put on the cake.

3 Cut the jelly snakes
  to make the hands
of the clock, pointing
them to the child's age.
Put the freckle in the
centre of the cake.

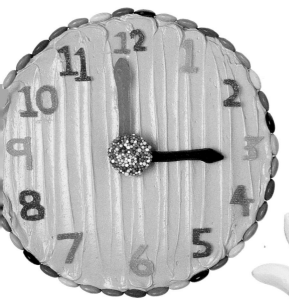

Index